CW00839117

LIVING WELL WITH LONG TERM CONDITIONS

Getting involved in the decisions that matter to you the most

Dr Gayathri Dittakavi
MRCGP,MBBS

Copyright © Dr Gayathri Dittakavi 2019

The right of Dr Gayathri Dittakavi to be identified as the author of this work has been asserted by him/her in accordance with the Copyright, Designs and Patents Act 1988

All rights reserved. This book is sold subject to the condition that no part of this book is to be reproduced, in any shape or form. Or by way of trade, stored in a retrieval system or transmitted in any form or by any means, electronic, mechanical, photocopying, recording, be lent, re-sold, hired out or otherwise circulated in any form of binding or cover other than that in which it is published and without a similar condition, includ-ing this condition being imposed on the subsequent purchaser, without prior permission of the copyright holder.

Cover Design and Typesetting by www.bookstyle.co.uk

Printed in Maya Printers, Bengaluru

A CIP catalogue record for this book is available from the British Library

ISBN - 978-1-9161607-0-5

FOREWORD

I am pleased to introduce this book written by Gayathri, who did her GP training with us at Gilberdyke Health Centre. During her time with us, Gayathri developed the skills to become a competent and patient centred GP. I think her writing this book is an extension of the enthusiasm she feels in caring for her patients and wanting them to get the best possible medical care that they can.

During long term condition reviews in General practice, we would like to be able to spend more time with you to discuss the many issues which are relevant to your care. But due to various constraints, this is not always possible. Information is given in small amounts at different times. The purpose of this book is to provide you with all the information that you need in simple terms and in one place.

When come to your review, having read the book, you will be able to feel confident in discussing the topics that matter to you the most at that particular time and if you need further information then you can always refer back to the book at a later date. Getting involved in the decision-making process will empower you to get the healthcare which meets your preferences and beliefs.

This book helps you guide through various pertinent topics like healthy lifestyle, social care and legal aspects of your health which are essential in planning your future care with excellent links to further information if needed.

Living with long term conditions can be challenging and when you fully engage in the decision-making process it helps us deliver the best care for you. This is something that we strive to achieve every day. Looking back at the thousands of consultations we have done, working in partnership with patients has always provided better outcomes, which is both satisfying to you and to us.

Dr Tanya Webb
General Practitioner
Gilberdyke Health Centre.

INTRODUCTION

Many adults have one or more long-term conditions for which there is no specific cure, but which can be managed with a combination of lifestyle changes and medications. As a general practitioner meeting with these patients for review of their condition(s), I have spent much time looking for good sources of information I could give them to take away that was simple to understand and covered a range of relevant topics. There is a lot of useful information online but many of my patients are unable to access it. They would still prefer a book or other printed material to read and reflect on, in their own time. Hence the idea for this book was conceived.

HOW TO USE THIS BOOK

If you have a long-term condition, it will need to be monitored regularly to prevent any problems arising from the condition. Discussing your condition with your doctor or nurse will help you to understand how to best manage it by making changes to your lifestyle and taking the medication you have been prescribed. There is a lot of evidence that regular review and good control of long-term conditions improve patients' outcomes and quality of life.

This book has been written to help you start discussions with your doctor or nurse regarding your long-term medical condition(s) and their management.

Consultations for review of long-term medical conditions can be challenging, especially if you have more than one condition. Although it may be difficult to discuss all the relevant information at the same time, this book can act as a guide to help you discuss the topics that concern you at any given time. Take it along to your reviews to help you raise the questions that are most important for you.

Having one or more long-term conditions should not stop you from living to your full potential. Improving your understanding of your condition(s) and how the health-care system works to support you will help to prevent misunderstandings on both sides. This book focuses on self-care and empowering you to get more involved in the decisions that matter most to you. It provides ideas about how to take control of your future health care and will help you to make health-care professionals aware of your thoughts and desires. They can then tailor your treatments to your wishes and beliefs and provide personalized care.

You can also discuss the topics with your close family members, friends and others involved with your care. This will help them to feel confident in supporting you.

There is also a lot of information on the internet and links to further sources of relevant and reliable information are provided at the end of each topic. There is also space for you to write information about locally available resources for each topic, for your future reference.

ACKNOWLEDGEMENTS

I dedicate this book to my dearest parents and brothers, because of whom I am a doctor. I cannot thank them enough for their love, dedication and sacrifices they have made for me, which has brought out the best in me. Your blessings are my strength.

My heartfelt thanks go to my dear husband for all his support, advice and unrelenting encouragement. You have always had my best interests at heart. Many thanks also to Bhargav, my lovely son, who is a great motivator.

I am grateful to Dr Webb and Dr Brotherton, my trainers at Gilberdyke Health Surgery, for proofreading this book and giving their valuable suggestions.

My sincere thanks go to all the teachers, who have taught me worthwhile lessons throughout my life.

Very special thanks are extended to my good friend, Dr Vinod Sanem, who is a pain consultant at Hull Royal Infirmary, and to Dr Dawn Moody, a GP who specializes in frailty, for taking time out from their busy schedules to give me their expert opinion on relevant topics.

Thanks also to our lovely friend Barbara and her friends for giving their invaluable comments after reading the draft copy.

I would like to thank Penny Howes for her excellent editing of the book and Charlotte Mouncey for creating a wonderful design for the book.

Last but not least, I must express my eternal gratitude to the patients who have been my true inspiration to write this book.

As my son says, we do best as a TEAM – Together we Achieve More – the soul of this book.

CONTENTS

CLINICAL CONDITIONS

LIFESTYLE MANAGEMENT

SOCIAL CARE

END-OF-LIFE CARE AND LEGAL ASPECTS

OTHER TOPICS RELATED TO YOUR HEALTH AND WELL-BEING

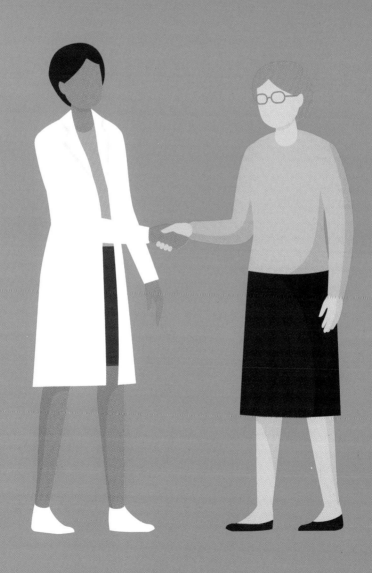

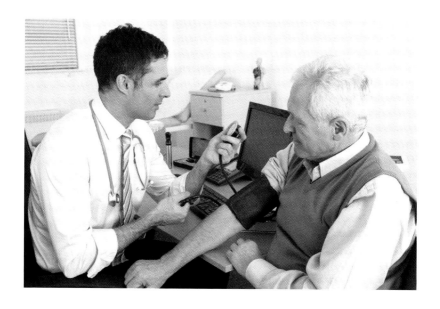

DIABETES

Diabetes means that you cannot control the levels of sugar in your blood.

 CAUSES

Insulin is a hormone that controls the levels of sugar in your blood. It is produced by a gland called the pancreas. If you have diabetes, your pancreas does not produce enough insulin and so you cannot control the amount of sugar in your blood after a meal.

 SYMPTOMS

- Tiredness

- Weight loss or weight gain

- Excessive thirst or needing to urinate more often

- Blurred vision

- Tingling or numbness in the hands and feet

- You may also get more infections such as colds and flu

MANAGEMENT

 Diagnosis

Your doctor can diagnose diabetes from a blood test. You may be asked to fast before having the blood test. Fasting means not eating for about 8–10 hours (usually overnight). You can have water.

 Lifestyle changes

Maintaining a healthy lifestyle is a key factor in controlling your blood sugar levels well.

See the topics on Lifestyle management.

 Treatment

Unfortunately, there is no cure for diabetes, but it can be managed by making sure your blood sugar levels are well controlled.

If you need medical treatment for your diabetes, it will either be regular oral tablets or injections.

Your doctor/nurse will be able to discuss with you, which treatment is best for you, depending on your blood sugar levels and your general health.

COMPLICATIONS

If you are taking tablets or having injections for diabetes, a complication that can occur is low blood sugar (hypo-glycaemia). This may happen if you do not eat meals at regular times.

Symptoms include nausea, dizziness and shaking.

It can usually be treated as soon as symptoms start, by having some sugary food (e.g. a biscuit) or drink. If it is not treated, it can lead to collapse and coma and may be life-threatening.

Sometimes if you have diabetes and are also unwell with another condition, such as flu, your blood sugar levels can go very high (hyperglycaemia), making you feel more unwell.

Symptoms of hyperglycaemia are extreme thirst, increased frequency of urination and confusion/disorientation.

You must seek urgent medical attention if you have these symptoms.

It is important to control your diabetes well, to reduce the risk of serious complications such as stroke, heart attack, loss of vision, nerve pains or kidney failure.

Poorly controlled diabetes may also reduce the circulation to the fingers and toes. This may eventually cause gangrene, requiring amputation.

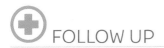 FOLLOW UP

It is important to have regular follow up with your doctor for blood pressure checks, blood tests, foot checks, medication reviews and mental health review.

It is also important to have regular eye checks with your optician, as diabetes can cause changes in the eyes that need to be picked up early.

USEFUL RESOURCES

- Diabetes UK (www.diabetes.org.uk)
- Check with your doctor for local resources

CHRONIC KIDNEY DISEASE

Chronic kidney disease means gradually worsening kidney disease that does not go away. It cannot be cured but can be managed to minimise the symptoms.

 ## CAUSES

The kidneys filter toxic substances out of the blood. If the kidneys do not work properly, these substances build up in the body and make you feel unwell.

High blood pressure, diabetes, high cholesterol, ageing, and some over-the-counter (e.g. ibuprofen, naproxen) or herbal medicines can cause chronic kidney disease.

 ## SYMPTOMS

- Tiredness

- Nausea (feeling sick or being sick)

- Hypertension (high blood pressure)

- Itching

- Swelling in the arms and legs

MANAGEMENT

 ### Diagnosis

Chronic kidney disease is diagnosed by doing blood and urine tests.

Depending on how bad the disease is, chronic kidney disease is classified as mild, moderate or severe.

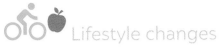 Lifestyle changes

You will probably need to make changes to your diet. A dietician will be able to help you with this.

Maintaining a healthy lifestyle with a good diet and regular exercise is important to help prevent and manage chronic kidney disease.

See the topics on Lifestyle management.

 Treatment

Many patients will not have any long-term problems and will only require monitoring of the condition.

If you have mild to moderate chronic kidney disease, your doctor will give you regular check-ups and may prescribe medicines to prevent worsening of your kidney function.

If you have severe chronic kidney disease, you will be referred to a specialist at the hospital, called a nephrologist. You may need dialysis.

Dialysis is an artificial way of removing toxic substance from your blood. A machine or a bag is connected to your abdomen and is used to filter your blood over several hours. Dialysis is usually done in the hospital as a day patient.

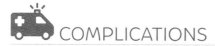 COMPLICATIONS

Chronic kidney disease increases your risk of having a heart attack or stroke.

If you become unwell with any of the symptoms listed on the previous page, you need to see your doctor urgently.

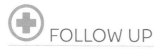 FOLLOW UP

It is important to have regular follow up with your doctor for blood pressure checks, blood tests, urine tests and medication reviews.

USEFUL RESOURCES

- NKF – Kidney Patients UK (www.kidney.org.uk)
- Check with your doctor for local resources

HYPERTENSION

Hypertension is high blood pressure.

 CAUSES

There are two types of hypertension:

- Essential hypertension, where no obvious cause can be found.

- Secondary hypertension is caused by other under-lying conditions such as thickening or narrowing of blood vessels, kidney disease or hormonal imbalance.

 SYMPTOMS

- There are no specific symptoms of hypertension.

- Very high blood pressure may cause headache, blurred vision, chest pain or palpitations.

MANAGEMENT

 Diagnosis

Hypertension is diagnosed by measurement of blood pressure over 24 hours or 7 days.

 Lifestyle changes

Hypertension can be greatly improved by following a healthy lifestyle.

Maintaining a healthy lifestyle with a good diet and regular exercise is important for good blood pressure control. It is especially important not to have too much salt in your diet.

See the topics on Lifestyle management.

 Treatment

Your doctor will be able to help you with choosing the right medication for you.

 COMPLICATIONS

Hypertension is a major risk factor for stroke, heart attack, eye disease and kidney failure.

 FOLLOW UP

It is important to have regular follow up with your doctor for blood pressure checks, blood tests, urine tests and medication reviews, and to have regular eye tests with your optician.

You can have a blood pressure machine at home and record your blood pressure at different times of the day. You can discuss this with your doctor when you attend for check-ups.

USEFUL RESOURCES

- British and Irish Hypertension Society (https://bihsoc.org/)
- Check with your doctor for local resources

ISCHAEMIC HEART DISEASE

Ischaemic heart disease (also known as coronary heart disease) includes a range of heart diseases, from mild angina to heart attack.

 ## CAUSES

Ischaemic heart disease is caused by blockage of the blood vessels of the heart.

Risk factors include:

- high cholesterol
- hypertension (high blood pressure)
- obesity
- smoking
- excess alcohol consumption
- diabetes
- age over 60 years
- family history of heart disease.

 ## SYMPTOMS

Symptoms depend on the degree of blockage of the blood vessels.

- Angina is chest pain that occurs on exertion or at rest.

- Heart attack means significant blockage of blood vessels. There may be severe chest pain but sometimes there is no pain at all. You may have other symptoms like generally feeling unwell, nausea (feeling or being sick), sweating or shortness of breath.

If you have chest pain lasting more than 10 minutes, call 999

MANAGEMENT

 Diagnosis

If you have chest pain sometimes, or all the time, you should see your doctor, who will arrange for you to have blood tests, an ECG (tracing of your heart's activity), a treadmill test, and a scan of your heart. This is called an angiogram – dye inserted through a vein travels to the heart, and imaging is then used to look for the blockage of the blood vessels.

 Lifestyle changes

Maintaining a healthy lifestyle with a good diet, plenty of exercises, stopping smoking and reducing alcohol consumption all help to prevent recurrence of the symptoms of ischaemic heart disease. See the topics on Lifestyle management.

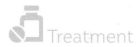
Treatment

Mild ischaemic heart disease can be treated with various medications.

You may need an angioplasty; this is a short surgical procedure where the blockage in the blood vessels to the heart is removed and a stent is inserted to keep the vessels open.

If there is a serious blockage, you will be considered for bypass surgery; a new section of the blood vessel is grafted to the blocked vessel, to "get around" the blockage.

COMPLICATIONS

Ischaemic heart disease can reduce your physical ability to do your activities.

It can also lead to symptoms of heart failure. These include shortness of breath on exertion, being unable to lay flat on a bed and swelling of legs; these symptoms are all due to fluid retention in the body.

FOLLOW UP

If you have had a heart attack, you will be offered cardiac rehabilitation. This is a programme to help you gradually get back to your normal activities.

It is important to have regular follow up with your doctor for blood pressure checks, blood tests and medication reviews, to prevent recurrence of ischaemic heart disease.

USEFUL RESOURCES

- British Heart Foundation – Coronary heart disease (https://www.bhf.org.uk/informationsupport/conditions/coronary-heart-disease)

- British Heart Foundation – Heart failure (https://www.bhf.org.uk/informationsupport/conditions/heart-failure)

- Check with your doctor for local resources

ATRIAL FIBRILLATION

Atrial fibrillation is a heart condition, where your heart-beat is irregular. This predisposes you to the formation of clots in the heart, which can travel to the brain and cause stroke.

 CAUSES

Causes include ageing, heart disease, hypertension (high blood pressure), thyroid imbalance, infections and salt imbalances.

Smoking, excess caffeine or alcohol consumption and obesity are known risk factors.

 SYMPTOMS

Very often atrial fibrillation is not associated with any symptoms, though you may have one or more of the symptoms listed below.

• Palpitations

• Chest tightness or pains

• Shortness of breath

• Dizziness

MANAGEMENT

Diagnosis

Atrial fibrillation is diagnosed by an irregular pulse or heartbeat on examination. This will then be checked with an ECG (tracing of your heart's activity) and blood tests.

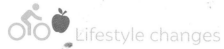

Lifestyle changes

Maintaining a healthy lifestyle with a good diet and regular exercise prevents worsening of the condition and complications. See the topics on Lifestyle management.

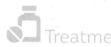

Treatment

Treating the underlying cause can sometimes stop the irregular heartbeat.

Medications may be used to help reduce the heart rate and/or to thin the blood so that clots are not formed.

You may have heard of medications like warfarin, which is used to thin your blood. Other newer medications like rivaroxaban and apixaban are also used.

If you need other treatments or procedures, they will be suggested by a heart specialist.

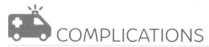

COMPLICATIONS

Possible complications include stroke and heart failure.

If you are on blood-thinning drugs, you may bleed

easily, so you will need to be assessed promptly if you have an injury.

Your prescribed medications may interact with over-the-counter drugs, so you should discuss this with your doctor.

 FOLLOW UP

It is important to have regular follow up with your doctor for blood pressure checks, blood tests and medication reviews, to prevent complications.

USEFUL RESOURCES

- British Heart Foundation – Atrial fibrillation (AF), causes, symptoms, diagnosis and treatment (https://www.bhf.org.uk/informationsupport/conditions/atrial-fibrillation)

- AF Association (www.atrialfibrillation.org.uk)

- National Institute for Health and Care Excellence – patient decision aid to help choose medications (https://www.nice.org.uk/guidance/cg180/resources/patient-decision-aid-pdf 243734797)

- Check with your doctor for local resources

STROKE

Stroke is when the blood supply to part of the brain is cut off. It is a medical emergency.

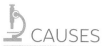 CAUSES

There are two types of stroke:

- Ischaemic stroke, when a blood clot blocks the flow of blood and oxygen to the brain; this is the most common type of stroke.

- Haemorrhagic stroke, when a blood vessel bursts and bleeds into the brain.

Causes include ischaemic heart disease, high cholesterol, hypertension (high blood pressure), diabetes, smoking, excess alcohol consumption, family history of aneurysms and irregular heartbeat.

 SYMPTOMS

Symptoms depend on whether blockage of the blood vessels is complete or only partial, or on the amount of bleeding, and which part of the brain is affected. They include the following:

- facial droop

- speech disturbance

- weakness on one side of the body

- dizziness

- double vision.

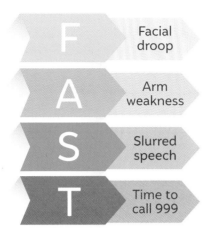

MANAGEMENT

 Diagnosis

If you have mild symptoms, you will need to see your doctor immediately and have blood tests, an ECG (tracing of your heart's activity), and scans of your brain, heart and blood vessels in your neck.

 Lifestyle changes

Maintaining a healthy lifestyle with a good diet and regular exercise is important for the prevention of further stroke. See the topics on Lifestyle management.

 Treatment

Your doctor/specialist will advise you on the medications you need, depending on your test results. You will need to be on long-term medications to help prevent complications.

If you have significant symptoms, you need to call an ambulance immediately and be seen as an emergency for treatment. This may involve medicines for thrombolysis (clot busting) or surgery.

 COMPLICATIONS

Serious stroke may result in severe physical and mental disability, speech and swallowing problems, visual disturbance, fits, dementia or death.

 FOLLOW UP

It is important to have regular follow up with your doctor for blood pressure checks and medication reviews, to prevent further strokes.

Your prescribed medications may interact with over-the-counter drugs (especially aspirin), so you should discuss this with your doctor.

After you have had a stroke, you may need rehabilitation to improve the strength in your muscles. This can vary from weeks to months or years. Physiotherapists and occupational therapists will help with your recovery. See the section on Social Care.

USEFUL RESOURCES

- Stroke Association (www.stroke.org.uk/)
- Check with your doctor for local resources

HYPERCHOLESTEROLAEMIA

Hypercholesterolaemia means high cholesterol in the blood. This condition may increase your risk of getting a heart attack, stroke, other vascular conditions or dementia.

 ## CAUSES

- Hypercholesterolaemia may be caused by consuming high quantities of foods that are high in fat, especially animal fat.

- It may also be linked to smoking or being inactive.

- It is more likely as you get older.

- In some people, it may be genetic and run in the family – there may be a family history of heart disease or stroke at a young age.

 ## SYMPTOMS

There are usually no specific symptoms, but you may have yellowish-white patches under your eyes, or around your joints.

MANAGEMENT

 ### Diagnosis

Hypercholesterolaemia is diagnosed with blood tests, and sometimes also genetic tests. Your doctor will test your blood for total, "good" and "bad" cholesterol and triglycerides.

Your doctor will use a tool called QRISK2 to calculate your risk of having a heart attack and stroke. This is used to help decide whether you need medications to reduce your cholesterol levels to prevent complications.

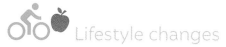 Lifestyle changes

Maintaining a healthy lifestyle with a good diet that is low in animal fats, regular exercise and weight reduction prevent worsening of the condition and complications. It is also important to take the medications your doctor suggests.

See the topics on Lifestyle management.

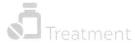 Treatment

You may be given tablets to reduce your cholesterol levels. These are called statins.

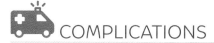 COMPLICATIONS

Complications include increased risk of heart attack, stroke, hypertension (high blood pressure) and dementia.

There are a lot of reports in the media about statins and this can be confusing. Statins should be prescribed according to your individual risks and it is important to discuss with your doctor what suits you best.

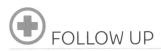 FOLLOW UP

It is important to have regular follow up with your doctor for blood tests. You may be asked to fast before having the blood test. Fasting means not eating for about 8–10 hours (usually overnight). You can have water.

If you are on statin tablets, you will also need regular blood tests and you need to know about interaction with other medications or some foods (e.g. you should not eat grapefruit or drink grapefruit juice). Your doctor can give you advice.

USEFUL RESOURCES

- British Heart Foundation (www.britishheart-foundation.org.uk); search for 'Cholesterol' and 'Hypercholesterolaemia'

- NHS – High cholesterol (www.nhs.uk/conditions/high-cholesterol/)

- National Institute for Health and Care Excellence (NICE), patient decision aid for taking statins; this is a useful tool to help you decide on the need to take statins (https://www.nice.org.uk/guidance/cg181/resources/patient-decision-aid-pdf-243780159)

- Check with your doctor for local resources

DEMENTIA

Dementia (for example, Alzheimer's dementia, vascular dementia, etc) is memory loss and confusion that affect your daily activities. It can vary from mild to severe.

 ## CAUSES

Dementia can be caused by the reduced blood supply to the brain, due to blockage of blood vessels, or by certain nerve conditions or some other unknown cause.

Memory impairment and confusion can also be caused by other conditions that are temporary. Once the underlying condition has been treated, memory improves. Examples are an infection, hormone imbalance, vitamin deficiency or salt imbalances.

 ## SYMPTOMS

Symptoms can occur gradually over a period of time and include forgetting things, confusion and changes in behaviour.

MANAGEMENT

 ### Diagnosis

If your doctor thinks you may have dementia, he or she will ask you to do a simple questionnaire to see how well you can remember information. This may be done at a memory clinic.

You will also have blood and urine tests and may also have a scan of your brain to check if there is an underlying cause that can be treated.

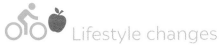

Lifestyle changes

Maintaining a healthy lifestyle with a good diet, regular exercise and plenty of social contacts may slow the progression of the symptoms of dementia. See the topics on Lifestyle management.

It is important to prepare for your future care if you lose the capacity to make decisions for yourself. This is discussed in more detail in the sections on Social care and End-of-life care and legal aspects.

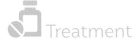

Treatment

Memory impairment can be daunting to you and your family and this can be a very worrying time.

There are many things that can be done to help you, especially if dementia is diagnosed early. Some medications started early can help to prevent the progression of the impairment.

Understanding and accepting the condition will help you and your family to prepare better for managing the condition. As dementia progresses, you may need more support and help from other professionals like nurses, carers, occupational therapists or physiotherapists. See the section on Social Care.

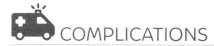

COMPLICATIONS

Memory impairment can lead to a gradual loss of independence, making you vulnerable to fraud or abuse (financial, physical or emotional), as well as self-neglect, which could affect your general health. It is important to make sure you have people you trust who can help you.

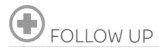

FOLLOW UP

It is important to have regular follow up with your doctor for blood pressure checks, blood tests, memory checks and medication reviews.

USEFUL RESOURCES

- Dementia UK (www.dementiauk.org)
- Check with your doctor for local resources

DEPRESSION

Depression means very low mood.

 CAUSES

Depression is caused by a reduction in certain chemicals in the brain. There may be no specific cause, but often depression results from a significant life event, such as bereavement, a change in physical health, or other change in circumstances, e.g. retirement, children leaving home, divorce.

 SYMPTOMS

Typical symptoms are low mood and feelings of low self-worth, hopelessness, sadness and no motivation to do your daily activities. Without treatment, depression may progress to neglecting yourself and thoughts of self-harm or even suicide.

MANAGEMENT

 Diagnosis

Your doctor can use the PHQ-9 questionnaire to find out the severity of your depression symptoms.

You may also have anxiety. Sometimes you can have anxiety along with depression, and the GAD questionnaire can be used to find out the severity of your anxiety symptoms.

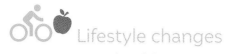 Lifestyle changes

Maintaining a healthy lifestyle will help you cope with symptoms better. It is important to try and have a regular daily routine, for example getting up and going to bed at the same time each day. A healthy diet, exercise, hobbies that interest you, and involvement in social activities are all positive coping mechanisms.

See the topics on Lifestyle management.

Drinking too much alcohol, smoking or taking illegal drugs can worsen your depression and should be avoided.

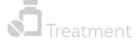 Treatment

It can be very difficult to talk about your feelings, but you should be confident that health professionals are there to help guide you to the treatment that is best for you.

You may be offered psychological therapies like counselling or cognitive behavioural therapy (CBT).

There is also an option of trying medications to help you. These are not addictive, but it is important to understand that it usually takes a few weeks for them to have any effect and a few months to see the full benefit, usually a minimum of 6 months.

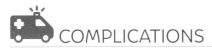

COMPLICATIONS

Risks of depression include - self-neglect, deterioration in general health, loneliness and becoming vulnerable to fraud or abuse (financial, physical or emotional).

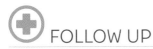

FOLLOW UP

It is important to have regular follow up with your doctor for medication reviews. Follow up with counsellors will improve your ability to cope long term.

USEFUL RESOURCES

- NHS – Clinical depression
  (www.nhs.uk/conditions/clinical-depression/)
- Mind (www.mind.org.uk)
- Age UK (www.ageuk.org.uk)
- Check with your doctor for local resources

PARKINSON'S DISEASE

Parkinson's disease is a progressive disorder of the brain that leads to disorders of movement.

 ## CAUSES

Parkinson's disease is caused by a reduction in a chemical in the brain called dopamine. Dopamine is important for movement.

 ## SYMPTOMS

- Involuntary shaking (tremors)

- Stiff muscles

- Slow movement, with a typical shuffling walk

- Taking more time than usual between deciding to move and actually being able to do so

MANAGEMENT

 ### Diagnosis

Parkinson's disease is diagnosed by clinical examination, usually with a specialist at a hospital. You will have blood tests and a brain scan.

 ### Lifestyle changes

Maintaining a healthy lifestyle with a good diet and regular exercise, as appropriate, will help you to cope with the disease better.

See the topics on Lifestyle management.

 Treatment

Depending on the degree of your symptoms, you will be offered treatment that is appropriate. There is no cure, but medications will delay progression and control your symptoms.

 COMPLICATIONS

You may experience depression, anxiety, balance problems, changes in your blood pressure or problems with smell, sleep and memory.

 FOLLOW UP

You will need to attend for regular follow up with the specialist for specific treatments. Specialist Parkinson's nurses will support your care.

It is also important to see your own doctor regularly for general health advice to help manage your condition better.

USEFUL RESOURCES

- Parkinson's UK (www.parkinsons.org.uk)
- Check with your doctor for local resources

OSTEOPOROSIS

Osteoporosis is weakening of the bones.

 CAUSES

- Low calcium and vitamin D; this may be caused by not having enough calcium in your diet and/or lack of exposure to sunlight
- Certain medications such as steroids
- Hormonal imbalances
- Ageing
- Lack of exercise, especially weight-bearing exercise
- Family history of brittle bones

 SYMPTOMS

Fractures resulting from very minor falls or injuries.

MANAGEMENT

 Diagnosis

Your doctor will assess your risk of osteoporosis using the Fracture Risk Assessment Tool (FRAX). This is a questionnaire that uses details such as your height and weight and asks about your lifestyle and family history.

You will have blood tests done and a DEXA scan (bone scan) will help to find out whether you have brittle bones.

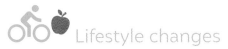 Lifestyle changes

Maintaining a healthy lifestyle with a good diet and regular exercise prevents worsening of the condition and reduces complications. It is particularly important to do weight-bearing exercise.

See the topics on Lifestyle management.

 Treatment

If you are at risk of osteoporosis or have brittle bones, your doctor will probably suggest that you take calcium and vitamin D supplements.

There are a few other medications that can help prevent the progression of brittle bones. Your doctor will prescribe them if you need them.

 COMPLICATIONS

If you have osteoporosis, you are at particular risk of bone fractures, especially of the hip and spine. This can cause significant disability and loss of independence.

 FOLLOW UP

It is important to have regular follow up with your doctor for blood tests and medication reviews. You should also have a DEXA scan at regular intervals.

USEFUL RESOURCES

- Royal Osteoporosis Society (https://nos.org.uk)
- Check with your doctor for local resources

ARTHRITIS

Arthritis is generally known as wear and tear of the joints.

 CAUSES

Arthritis is usually part of the ageing process. There is a reduction of fluid and space in your joints, which causes pain and swelling.

 SYMPTOMS

- Pain, swelling or crackling sound in the joint
- Locking of the joint
- Joint giving way
- Stiffness in the joint

MANAGEMENT

 Diagnosis

Diagnosis is mainly by clinical examination. X-rays and scans can be used to check the severity of arthritis but are not always needed.

 Lifestyle changes

Maintaining a healthy lifestyle by reducing your weight and staying as active as possible will help reduce pain and improve your mobility.

See the topics on Lifestyle management.

Mobility aids will help build your confidence to move and prevent you from falling.

 Treatment

Pain can be controlled by painkillers. Your doctor can advise you on which one is best for you.

Physiotherapy and regular exercises will help to strengthen the muscles around the affected joint, reduce your symptoms and improve your mobility.

You may be referred to a specialist orthopaedic doctor, who can help you decide whether joint replacement is right for you.

 COMPLICATIONS

The main risks associated with arthritis are limited mobility with reduced activities and loss of independence. This can lead to poor general health and self-care. There is also an increased risk of falls.

Inappropriate use of painkillers can also cause harmful side-effects and other complications.

 FOLLOW UP

It is important to have regular follow up with your doctor for medication reviews and to check whether your arthritis is progressing.

You should be able to self-manage your pain.

See the topic of Pain control.

USEFUL RESOURCES

- Arthritis Research UK – a very good resource for self-management of arthritis (https://www.arthritisresearchuk.org)
- Check with your doctor for local resources

FREQUENT FALLS

Older people are at increased risk of falls that can seriously affect their mobility and impair their independence.

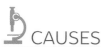 CAUSES

There are many possible causes and many falls are caused by a combination of factors. Some of these are listed next.

- Weakness in the limbs, or brain conditions, e.g. Parkinson's disease

- Joint pains

- Vision or hearing disturbance

- Heart conditions or low blood pressure

- Abnormalities in salt levels

- Some medications

- Ageing/frailty

MANAGEMENT

 Diagnosis

Your doctor will carry out a falls assessment to find out the cause of your falls.

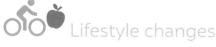 Lifestyle changes

Occupational therapists and physiotherapists will be able to guide you to make changes at home to help prevent falls. They can also help you with different aids, such as a walking frame, or handrails. See the topics on Social Care.

 Treatment

Treating the underlying cause of your falls should reduce your risk of falling again.

 COMPLICATIONS

Falls can lead to significant physical injuries like bone fracture or head injury. This, in turn, can lead to a loss of confidence in getting up and moving around, with loss of independence. It may also result in poor general health because of poor self-care.

 FOLLOW UP

It is important to have regular follow up with your doctor for blood pressure checks and medication reviews, to prevent more falls. It is also important to have regular eye checks with your optician and hearing checks with a hearing specialist.

USEFUL RESOURCES

- NHS – Falls (https://www.nhs.uk/conditions/ Falls/)
- Check with your doctor for local resources

ASTHMA AND CHRONIC OBSTRUCTIVE PULMONARY DISEASE (COPD)

Asthma is a common lung condition that is due to inflammation of the airways. COPD is a long-term lung condition due to damage to the airways and/or the air sacs in the lungs. Both conditions cause difficulties with breathing.

 CAUSES

There is no single known cause of asthma, but inflammation of the airways can be caused by allergens, pollution or infections. A family history of allergies can make you more prone to asthma.

COPD can be due to lifelong smoking, or long-term exposure to dust, chemicals or smoke, possibly at work.

A small number of people have an inherited deficiency of an enzyme called alpha-1 antitrypsin that helps to protect the lungs from damage. This makes them more susceptible to the effects of smoke and chemicals and to developing COPD.

 SYMPTOMS

- Asthma causes cough, wheeze and shortness of breath, usually from a young age. These often come on at night-time and can be very alarming. The symptoms are intermittent and reversible, usually by using an inhaler.

- COPD is a progressive disease and the symptoms are shortness of breath and cough, often with sputum (phlegm) production.

MANAGEMENT

 Diagnosis

Your doctor will be able to do some tests to find out which condition you have. You may have a chest X-ray and breathing tests to check your lung function.

 Treatment

There are many types of inhalers that can be used to help with your symptoms. Your doctor will prescribe the one that is best for you. You may also be given medications to help if your symptoms are worse.

If you are very poorly with your condition, you will be offered a nebulizer, breathing machine or oxygen to use at home.

 Lifestyle changes

It is important to avoid triggers for asthma.

Stopping smoking – It is never too late to stop smoking and there is lots of help available to quit smoking.

See the topic of Smoking – Lifestyle management.

If you use an inhaler, it is important to carry it with you at all times, in case of a sudden asthma attack.

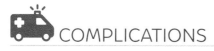 COMPLICATIONS

Asthma can be life-threatening – seek urgent medical help if your symptoms are worse or cannot be managed with your inhaler.

COPD can limit your mobility and activity, leading to a loss of independence. If your symptoms are not controlled well, you may need regular hospital admissions. It can sometimes lead to lung cancer.

 FOLLOW UP

It is important to have regular follow up with your doctor or nurse to check your lung function and your inhalers or medication, to help you control your symptoms and prevent worsening of your condition.

Annual flu vaccination and pneumococcal vaccination will prevent you from having significant chest infections.

USEFUL RESOURCES

- Asthma UK (https://www.asthma.org.uk)
- British Lung Foundation – COPD (https://www.blf.org.uk/support-for-you/copd)
- Check with your doctor for local resources

CANCER

Cancer is a condition where the cells of a particular part of the body grow and multiply abnormally. It can often begin as benign lesions that are localised but may become malignant when it spreads to other parts of the body and is usually life-threatening.

 RISK FACTORS

- Smoking

- Alcohol consumption

- Genetic factors

- Ageing

- Sun exposure

- Exposure to radiation

- Exposure to some chemicals

- Certain viruses

- Poor diet

- Obesity

 SYMPTOMS

Common symptoms of any cancer are fatigue, lethargy and weight loss.

Symptoms of specific cancers are shown in the next table.

MANAGEMENT

 Diagnosis

Any lumps in the body that are changing and causing symptoms need to be checked urgently. You will be referred to specialist clinics to have urgent tests done. The doctors and specialists will explain the tests to you.

Tests used to diagnose specific cancers are listed in the table on page 58.

 Lifestyle changes

A diagnosis of cancer can be life-changing. Maintaining a healthy lifestyle can help you cope better with the condition and the treatments.

Things that you might need to consider regarding your future care and planning are discussed in other topics, especially Living with persistent pain, in the section Lifestyle management, and some topics in the sections on Social care and End-of-life care and legal aspects.

 Treatment

There are many treatments available, depending on the stage of your cancer. These include chemotherapy, radiotherapy and surgery. Cancer specialists will discuss your management plan with you.

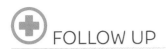 FOLLOW UP

You will be under the care of specialists and your own doctors. Do not hesitate to contact them if you have any doubts about your symptoms or treatment.

There might be many health professionals involved in your care and this can be daunting for you, but understanding who does what and feeling confident you are getting appropriate care will help you to cope better.

USEFUL RESOURCES

- Cancer Research UK (www.cancerresearchuk. org/)
- Macmillan cancer support (https://www.macmillan.org.uk)
- Check with your doctor for local resources

SYMPTOMS AND DIAGNOSIS OF SPECIFIC CANCERS

Cancer	Symptoms	Tests
Breast	Hard lump Change in size/ shape of the nipple Blood discharge from the nipple	Examination Scan Biopsy
Prostate/bladder	Urinary symptoms – difficulty urinating, or need to urinate more often Blood in urine	Prostate examination Blood test Biopsy Scan
Lung	Shortness of breath Persistent cough Coughing up blood	Chest X-ray Scan Bronchoscopy
Bowel	Change in bowel habit – alternate loose stool and constipation Blood or mucus in the stool Lump in the abdomen	Blood test Endoscopy – a camera test scan
Skin	Change in moles Changing or new skin lesions Itching/bleeding	Biopsy

Brain	Worsening headaches Weakness in limbs Speech/vision disturbance Dizziness Vomiting	Scan
Throat	Change in voice Cough Lump in the neck	Camera test Scan
Oesophagus	Difficulty in swallowing Chest discomfort Worsening reflux symptoms	Camera test Scan
Ovarian	Lump in the abdomen Bloating/distention of the abdomen Discomfort in the abdomen	Blood test Scan
Mouth	White patches Ulcers Lumps	Biopsy
Genital	New lesions/lumps Abnormal bleeding	Scan Biopsy

MALNUTRITION

In malnutrition, you are not getting the right amounts of nutrients, which leads to deterioration in your general health. There are two types of malnutrition: undernutrition (not enough food, or not enough of some nutrients) or over-nutrition (too much food – commonly known as obesity).

 ## CAUSES

Physical causes

- Long-term medical conditions
- Recurrent hospital admissions/deteriorating illness
- Reduced mobility and inability to prepare food
- Swallowing/gut problems
- Undereating or overeating
- Reduced exercise

Psychological causes

- Stress due to financial, family or work problems
- Social isolation or being in care

 ## SYMPTOMS

The main symptom of malnutrition is a significant change in your weight:

- Undernutrition: losing 5–10% of your weight over 3–6 months

- Overnutrition: gaining excessive weight

Other symptoms include excessive tiredness, falling ill frequently and taking longer periods to recover.

MANAGEMENT

 Diagnosis

You may notice changes to the size you need for clothes or jewellery, or your friends, family or health professionals may mention concerns.

Your nurse or doctor will measure your height and weight, and these are used to calculate your body mass index (BMI, measured in kg per m²) and work out whether you are underweight or overweight.

These are the values used:

below 18.5	you are in the underweight range
between 18.5 & 24.9	you are in the healthy weight range
between 25 & 29.9	you are in the overweight range
between 30 & 39.9	you are in the obese range

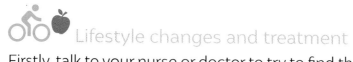 Lifestyle changes and treatment

Firstly, talk to your nurse or doctor to try to find the cause for the change in your weight. You could start by looking at the trend of your weight over the last few months and considering other things that have changed in that time.

If you are undernourished:

Depending on how underweight you are, your doctor, nurse or dietician can help guide you on what to eat and how much of it to eat.

- Commonly, you can have high-calories foods, fortified foods and over-the-counter supplements.

- Your doctor or dietician may suggest you take supplement drinks if you are severely undernourished.

- You may need support with your feeding by means of feeding tubes into your stomach. Alternatively, you could be given supplements through a drip inserted into one of your veins.

If you are overnourished or obese:

Depending on the cause, various interventions can be made to help you. Some are listed next.

- Looking into your food choices, portion sizes and lifestyle. Your nurse/doctor or dietician can help you with this.

- Discussing your activity levels and how they can be increased. You may be offered referral to local exercise programmes.

- Discussing your mental health issues and addressing them accordingly. Referral to a psychologist will help you achieve your targets better.

- Coping strategies with regard to social influences and making healthy choices even during difficult periods of life.

- Discussing with your doctor regarding medical conditions and medications causing you to gain weight and looking into alternative treatments.

- Joining local groups that support weight loss. Check with your nurse or doctor regarding locally available resources.

- If you are struggling with the above interventions, you may be considered for referral to a weight-management clinic, with the possibility of surgery.

Maintaining a healthy lifestyle with a good diet and regular exercise is important to help keep your weight at a healthy level.

See the topics on Lifestyle management.

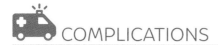 COMPLICATIONS

Undernutrition

- Reduced ability to carry out self-care and daily activities

- Recurrent infections due to reduced immunity, worsening your underlying long-term conditions

- Recurrent falls

- Social isolation, depression

- Deficiencies of micronutrients like iron, vitamin B_{12}, vitamin D or vitamin C can cause anaemia, brittle bones and bleeding problems.

Overnutrition or obesity

- Lots of studies have now shown that being over-weight or obese has adverse effects on many aspects of health.

- Being overweight or obese predisposes you to many of the conditions described in the previous topics in this section, especially heart conditions, stroke and diabetes. It can also make these conditions worse or more serious.

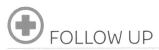 # FOLLOW UP

Regular follow up with your doctor, nurse or dietician can help you keep motivated in maintaining a healthy weight.

USEFUL RESOURCES

- British Nutrition Foundation – A healthy, balanced diet (https://www.nutrition.org.uk/ healthyliving/healthydiet/healthybalanced-diet.html)

- Check with your doctor, nurse or dietician for local resources on weight management

OTHER CONDITIONS THAT COMMONLY PRESENT WITH AGEING

Ageing is a process that none of us can avoid, but we can aim to stay active and healthy as long as possible. This topic presents information on some conditions that are common in older people.

EARS AND HEARING

Hearing loss can be a part of the ageing process and also other conditions like wax in the ear or infections in the ear.

Your doctor can refer you for a hearing test to find out the degree of hearing loss. You will be recommended to have hearing aids if you have problems hearing.

TEETH

It is important to have regular dental checks to maintain good dental hygiene.

FEET

It is important to look after your feet, especially if you suffer from long-term conditions such as diabetes or lack of mobility.

Podiatrists can help you with most issues of the feet.

Abnormal changes in the colour or sensations of your feet or cramps in the feet and legs need to be assessed by your doctor, as they may be a sign of an underlying condition.

SKIN

Dry skin and itching are common with ageing. They can be due to underlying medical conditions or to medications. Your doctor will be able to help with your symptoms.

INCONTINENCE

There are several possible causes for incontinence, and it may be caused by an underlying condition, so your doctor will want to investigate the reason. Incontinence of the bladder or bowel can be managed with incontinence pads, medications or surgery, depending on the cause.

USEFUL RESOURCES

- Age UK and NHS – A practical guide to healthy ageing (https://www.england.nhs.uk/wp-content/uploads/2019/04/a-practical-guide-to-healthy-ageing.pdf)
- Check with your doctor for local resources

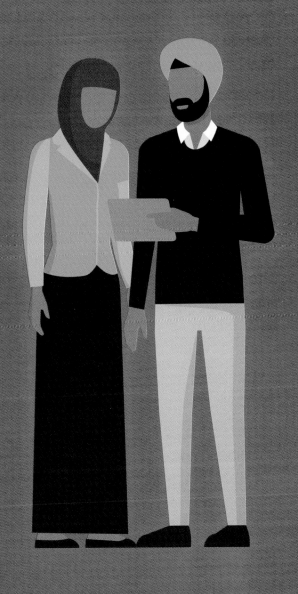

LIFESTYLE MANAGEMENT

It is important to have a healthy lifestyle throughout your life.

ENSURING A HEALTHY LIFESTYLE AS YOU GROW OLDER

As you grow older, your health and activity levels may change significantly and so you may need to think differently about how to stay healthy.

Depending on your general health, your doctor or nurse can give you recommendations regarding diet, exercise and other aspects of a healthy lifestyle.

Certain medical conditions need special recommendations. Maintaining a healthy lifestyle will help to prevent severe disabling complications/hospital admissions and loss of independence.

The topics in this section give you information about ways you can manage your lifestyle to stay as healthy as possible

HEALTHY DIET

A healthy diet means eating the right amount of a wide variety of foods so that you have enough energy for your activities and can maintain a healthy weight.

HOW MUCH FOOD DO I NEED?

Food is mainly made up of carbohydrates (source of sugar for energy), protein (helps build muscle), fats (store energy, insulate and protect organs), fibre, vitamins and minerals. When we consume food, it is converted into energy in our body.

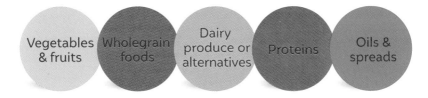

Your body needs energy for involuntary actions such as breathing and pumping blood around the body. It also needs energy for voluntary activities like walking, lifting, housework, gardening etc.

The energy in food is measured in calories. You need to have the right amount of calories each day for your involuntary and voluntary activities.

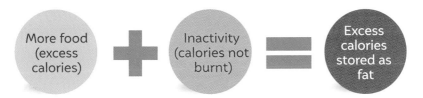

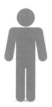

An average-built man with a good level of activity needs 2500 calories per day.

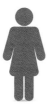

An average-built woman with a good level of activity needs 2000 calories per day.

SIMPLIFY YOUR DIET

It is important to eat three regular meals a day and to drink plenty of fluids each day.

Make a list of foods you like to eat.

Divide your foods depending on the calories and fat/protein/carbohydrate content.

Divide them as:

have these foods more often	
have these foods intermittently	
have these foods rarely or if possible, avoid.	

Make meal plans that are healthy and suit your diet and taste.

Once in a while, you can reward yourself for following a healthy diet.

You will start to notice significant improvements in your energy levels with a healthy diet.

Once a change is noticed, it becomes a habit, one that is difficult to break.

When you have a long-term medical condition, you might have to change your diet according to the illness and medications you need. Consult your doctor/nurse/ dietician regarding these changes.

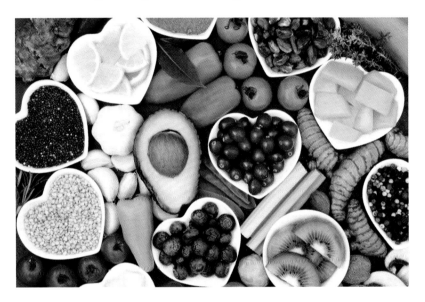

FACTORS THAT INFLUENCE EATING HABITS

Positive influences – spend time to increase these influences

- General good health
- Active lifestyle
- Social contact
- Stimulating activities

Negative influences – address these influences and find coping mechanisms

- Significant stressful life events
- Feeling unwell with medical conditions
- Peer pressure
- Low mood
- Inactivity
- Challenging work or social circumstances

USEFUL RESOURCES

- British Nutrition Foundation (www.nutrition.org.uk)
- Check with your doctor for local resources

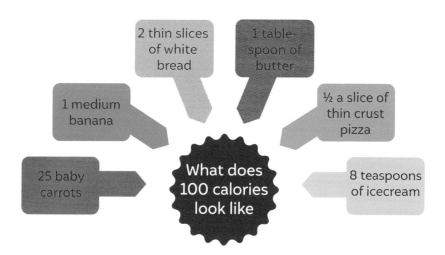

EXERCISE/ACTIVITY LEVELS

Even if you have a long-term condition, it is important for your physical and mental health to stay as active as possible.

WHAT ARE THE BENEFITS OF EXERCISE?

- Improved energy levels

- Better control of your medical conditions like hypertension (high blood pressure), high blood glucose levels

- Prevention of conditions like stroke, heart attack, complications of diabetes, high blood pressure, COPD

- Improvement in mobility, reduction in joint pains

- Maintaining a healthy weight

- Improvement in your mood

HOW MUCH- EXERCISE DO I NEED?

Recommendations for an average adult are at least

- 30 minutes per day

- 5 days per week

Activities include ordinary daily activities (such as house-work or gardening), structured exercise or sport, or a combination of these activities.

Tailor activities according to your general health, interests and personal circumstances.

INTENSITY OF EXERCISE

The level of activity and intensity can be classified as follows:

Inactive	a sedentary occupation and no physical exercise or cycling
Moderately inactive	a sedentary occupation and some but less than 1 hour of physical exercise and/or cycling per week, OR a standing occupation and no physical exercise or cycling
Moderately active	a sedentary occupation and 1–2.9 hours of physical exercise and/or cycling per week, OR a standing occupation and some but less than 1 hour of physical exercise and/or cycling per week, OR a physical occupation and no physical exercise or cycling
Active	a sedentary occupation and 3 hours or more of physical exercise and/or cycling per week, OR a standing occupation and 1–2.9 hours of physical exercise and/or cycling per week, OR a physical occupation and some but less than 1 hour of physical exercise and/or cycling per week, OR a heavy manual occupation.

0	Breathing easily, conversation easy
1	Breathing lightly and talking easily but heart rate increases
2	Still talking comfortably but breathing quickly and body warming up
3	Breathing more deeply and harder, talking with a little more difficulty
4	Breathing very hard and short of breath, cannot carry out a conversation

Light activity 0–1
Moderate activity 2–3
Vigorous activity 4

To be considered as moderate activity, walking should be 2–3.

If you are frail, you may need help with your activities, such as aids to help with your mobility.

Discuss with your nurse or doctor how you can improve your levels of activity safely.

There may be local services available on referral to help you with your activities.

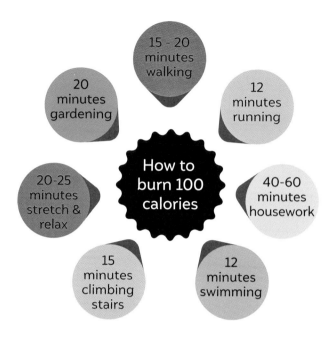

WHAT FACTORS WILL INFLUENCE MY LEVEL OF ACTIVITY?

Positive influences

- The benefits of general well-being

- Improvement in medical conditions

- Improved mood

- Good social support

Negative influences

- Poor health, leading to low energy levels

- Loneliness

- Smoking and excess alcohol consumption

- Significant stressful life events

- Feeling unwell with medical conditions

- Challenging work or social circumstances

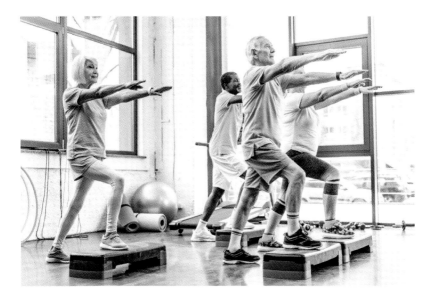

USEFUL RESOURCES

- NHS – Exercise
  (https://www.nhs.uk/live-well/exercise/)

- Check with your doctor for local resources

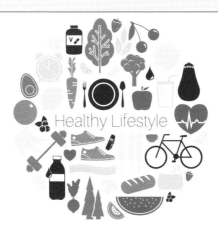

SMOKING

Smoking has a significant adverse effect on health for almost all the clinical conditions discussed in the Clinical conditions section.

It is never too late to stop smoking.

There are lots of options available to help you stop smoking, like nicotine products and other medications. Speak to your pharmacist, nurse or doctor regarding locally available stop smoking clinics.

There is evidence that, with help and support, your chances of quitting smoking over a long period of time are improved.

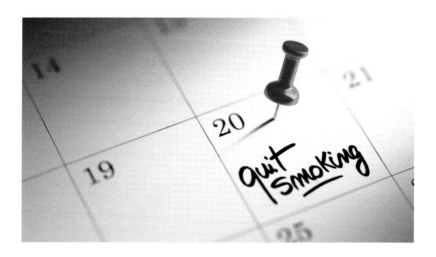

ALCOHOL CONSUMPTION

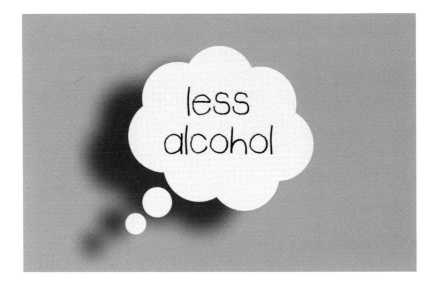

It is very important to know the safe limits of alcohol intake. Medication and alcohol don't usually go well together.

If you are drinking more than recommended and need help with stopping, you can be referred to a local centre to support withdrawal. Your nurse or doctor can help you with this information.

Recommended Safe Units per week
For Men and Women: 14 Units

Units of alcohol	Examples	Comments
1 UNIT	• ½ pint of standard lager, beer or cider • ½ pint of standard alcopop • 1 small glass of standard wine • 25 ml of standard whiskey (5 teaspoons)	*Knowing how many units helps you understand if you are drinking above safe limits*
2 UNITS	• 1-pint standard lager, beer or cider • 1 standard glass of standard wine or champagne • A double measure of spirit	*Check your labels for units*
3 UNITS	• 1 pint of higher strength lager, beer or cider • 1 large glass of lower strength wine	*Spread the 14 units of alcohol over more than 3 days*
10 UNITS	• 1 bottle of wine	*Many online tools and apps are available to calculate how much you drink*

SLEEP

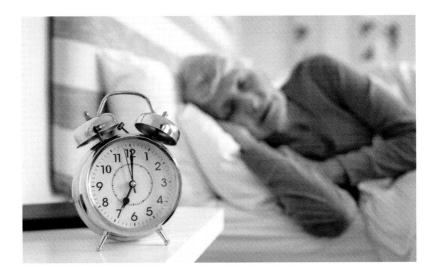

Sleep can be disturbed for various reasons and this can have adverse effects on your general health or health condition. It can be due to physical or mental health issues. If you need help, discuss with your doctor how you can improve your sleeping.

HELPFUL SLEEPING HABITS

- Having a set time to sleep and wake up that is the same every day

- Activities that help with your sleep, e.g. relaxation techniques, reading, having a bath

- Addressing your worries and concerns – you may need help from your doctor

- Avoiding caffeine, alcohol and smoking before going to bed, as these inhibit undisturbed sleep

- Not using a mobile phone or other screens in the bedroom

- Making an environment that encourages sleep – examples include optimum temperature, peaceful décor, a bed that is comfortable

USEFUL RESOURCES

- NHS – Sleep and tiredness (https://www.nhs.uk/live-well/ sleep-and-tiredness/how-to-get-to-sleep/)

EXTREME WEATHER CONDITIONS

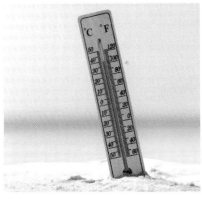 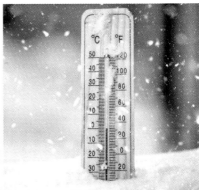

As you get older, it is harder to keep warm when it is cold or to cool down when it is hot. This poses some challenges for self-care in very cold or very warm temperatures.

HOT WEATHER

It is best to stay in the shade wherever possible and to use sunscreen if you are out in the sun. You also need to make sure you drink plenty of fluids.

Signs of heat stroke, which mean you urgently need to cool down, are:

- headache

- dizziness and confusion

- loss of appetite

- feeling sick

- excessive sweating

- pale, clammy skin

- cramps in the arms, legs and stomach

- fast breathing or pulse

- intense thirst

- a temperature of 38°C or above.

If you feel unwell outdoors, it is a good idea to go indoors and open the windows or use a fan to create a breeze. You could also have a cool bath to help you cool down.

COLD WEATHER

When it is very cold outside, you should try to keep your heating turned on all day. It is a good idea to use a room thermometer to check the temperature, which should be around 20°C. It is better to use several layers of clothing, rather than just one thick jumper.

Signs of hypothermia, which mean you urgently need to warm up, are:

- shivering

- cold and pale skin

- slurred speech

- fast breathing

- tiredness

- confusion, which may lead to collapse.

If you are very cold, a warm bath may be helpful.

MAKING CHANGES TO YOUR LIFESTYLE

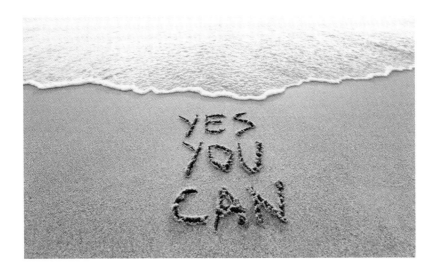

If you have a long-term condition, you will probably need to adopt some aspects of your lifestyle to cope with the changes that are forced on you. It is better to find ways to adapt rather than to "fight" issues that you cannot actually do anything about.

Changing your lifestyle can be challenging, as habits are often developed over many years. If you understand and accept why you need to change, that may make it easier, but it may still take some time to adapt.

THE CYCLE OF CHANGE

Understanding the stages of the cycle of change can help you understand where you are on the pathway to change and how to progress. The stages are listed in the diagram on the following page.

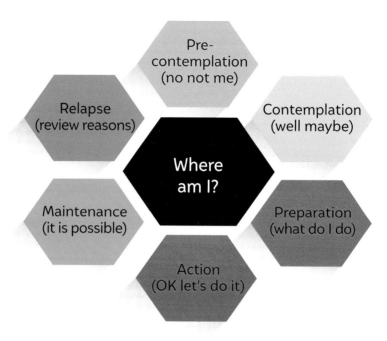

If you are trying to make a change, discuss with your nurse or doctor what stage you are at and what support you can get to help change a habit that is bad for your health.

MOTIVATIONAL INTERVIEWING FOR CHANGING A HABIT

It can also be helpful to use a motivational interview to help you make a change, such as changing your diet, improving your level of exercise or giving up smoking or drinking alcohol. An example of a motivational interview is given on the following page. Try writing down your answers to the questions to discuss with your nurse.

		Your answers
1.	What is the habit? Why is it a habit? Can it change?	
2.	What are the pros and cons of changing the habit?	
3.	What positive and negative impacts does the habit have on your health?	
4.	How can changes be made?	
5.	Were changes made before? How successful were you? Did you relapse? Why?	
6.	How will your future be if the habit is changed? Do you have any specific goals you want to achieve?	
7.	On a scale of 1 to 10, how important is your health? Why is it that number? What can be done to improve?	

MEDICATION COMPLIANCE

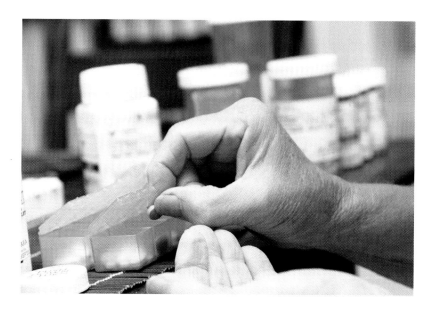

Medication compliance is correctly following the advice you have been given about when and how to take your prescribed medication.

WHY YOU MIGHT NOT BE COMPLIANT WITH YOUR MEDICATION

There are several reasons why a patient might not be compliant with medication. Some of these are listed next.

- Not understanding why a medication has been prescribed, believing it is not needed, or having some other concerns about the medication

- Forgetting to take the medication; this could be for several different reasons, such as:

  work

  stress

  memory impairment

  too many medications to take, often at different times of day

  side-effects of medications

  confusion about various forms of the medication (e.g. tablets/liquid medicine/patches)

- Depending on others to give you medications because of physical or memory impairments

- News articles giving contradictory messages about a particular medication and/or the opinions of family and friends

- The cost of medications

- Errors at the pharmacy, or in collecting or reordering prescriptions at the correct time

WHAT COULD HAPPEN IF I AM NON-COMPLIANT WITH MY MEDICATION?

Non-compliance with your prescribed medication can lead to worsening of your condition. This may mean treatment has to be stepped up, which could put you at more risk of becoming seriously ill.

WHAT SHOULD I DO IF I HAVE DIFFICULTY BEING COMPLIANT WITH MY MEDICATION?

It is important that you take all the medications your doctor has prescribed, even if you seem to have a lot to remember. If you have several different conditions that are being treated, it is especially important to take your medications at the right time of day to prevent side-effects or interactions between the different medications.

- Discuss with your doctor, nurse or pharmacist why the medication is prescribed, and keep asking questions until you are sure; it may help to write it down to help you remember.

- Make sure you understand what your options are and choose what is best for you while respecting what the doctor tells you that you need.

- Make sure you have regular medication reviews, and blood tests if you need them, especially if you are on multiple medications. Keep reminders for yourself of when you need to attend for review.

- You can use aids like blister packs, dossett boxes, a diary or a log book to help make sure you take all your medications at the right time of day.

See the topic Personal log book.

- If you are still having trouble, ask a relative or friend to help you.

LIVING WITH PERSISTENT PAIN

PAIN MEASUREMENT SCALE

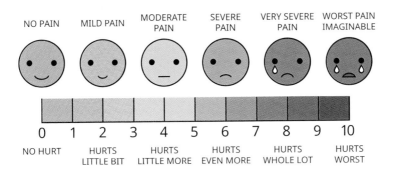

It can be challenging to manage persistent pain, but there are things you can do to help you cope and achieve a reasonable quality of life.

- Try to understand your pain and the activities that aggravate it; can these activities be done in small chunks, at a slower pace?

- Score your pain from 1 to 10, with 10 being the worst, and keep a diary to note any trends and help you to find out what may make it worse or better.

- Persistent pain can remain at the same level, gradually worsen, or have a waxing and waning progression. Try to tailor your activities accordingly.

- Accepting a certain level of pain and distracting or shifting focus on to other activities can be very helpful.

- Continue to be active, as this improves the threshold of pain. It will also improve your general health and mood, which in turn will help you cope better with pain.

- Taking optimum levels of rest during activities and trying to sleep if you need to will boost your energy levels.

- Mild to moderate levels of pain can be helped using painkillers as and when needed, along with the above recommendations. Make sure you let your doctor/nurse know about what you are using, as it is important to make sure that it is safe for you.

- If your pain score is high, you may need regular painkillers. Discuss with your doctor what your options are. Make sure you know how long you need to be on them. It is important to understand that at some point you will probably need to try and wean yourself off them if you no longer need them.

- Some groups of medication are addictive and it can be difficult to wean off them. You may be offered specialist help to try and stop.

- Make sure you are aware of the side-effects of these medications, both short term and long term. If you are taking any new medications check whether there are any drug interactions.

- Your doctor may refer you to a pain specialist, who may offer other options like injections or surgical interventions to help with your pain.

BLOOD TESTS AND FOLLOW UP

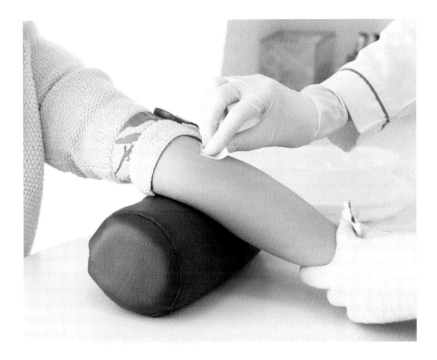

If you have one or more long-term conditions, you will probably need regular follow up, and possibly also regular blood tests. This is important to:

- monitor the progress of your condition
- pick up and treat any complications early
- make sure your medications are not having any adverse effects.

You may have blood tests done more often when your condition is first diagnosed and/or any medication is started or changed. Once the condition is stabilised, they can be done less often, perhaps 6-monthly or annually.

Your doctor or nurse can help you with this.

You may be asked to fast before having the blood test. Fasting means not eating for about 8–10 hours (usually overnight). You can have water.

If you are having tests done regularly, it is hard to remember when you are due next. You will find it helpful to keep a diary and respond to reminders sent from your doctor.

Discuss with your nurse/doctor what blood tests you are having done and why. You can discuss the results and what they mean for you, at a follow-up appointment.

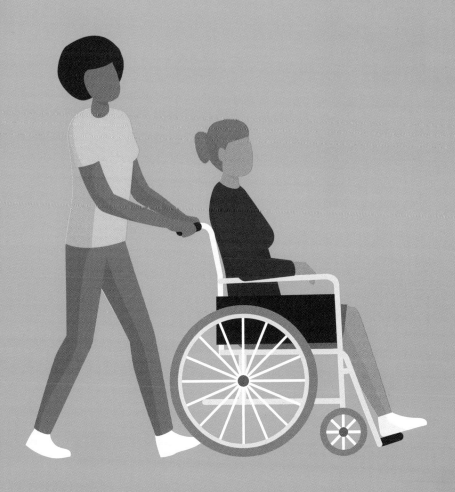

LIVING INDEPENDENTLY AT HOME

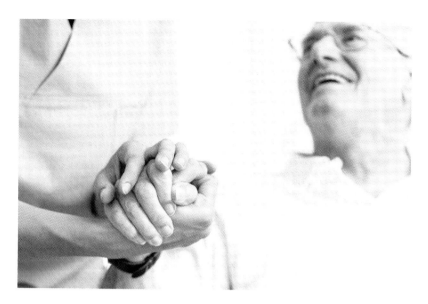

It is important to live at home and stay independent for as long as possible. You may need additional help or support to do this, especially if you have several long-term conditions. This section gives information about the support that is available to you.

CARERS

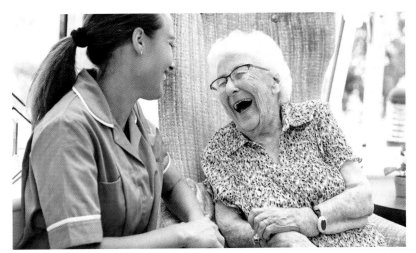

You may need a carer if you have difficulty caring for yourself, for example, because of illness, disability or general infirmity.

You may be a carer to someone who has difficulty caring for themselves.

IF YOU HAVE A CARER

- Make sure you both understand and agree with what your carer's roles are, and what they will and will not do. For example, you may initially only need help with getting to the shops or preparing meals, or just want company, but once you have a trusted carer or carers, this can progress to help with getting dressed and undressed, bathing, etc.

- Inform trusted family members and/or close friends that you have a carer or get them to help you find a suitable carer.

- Inform your doctor or nurse, as they may need to contact the carer for information or advice regarding your care.

- If you have any concerns, discuss them with a friend or family member who you trust, or with your doctor or nurse.

- Get help early if you have concerns.

IF YOU ARE A CARER

- Make sure you register yourself as a carer your local council to get more support. You may be eligible for financial support, pension credit, housing allowance or council tax reduction.

- You will need regular health checks yourself to ensure you stay healthy, as the other person is dependent on you.

FURTHER RESOURCES

- Carers UK (https://www.carersuk.org/)
- Public Health England – A practical guide to healthy caring (https://www.england.nhs.uk/wp-content/uploads/2016/04/nhs-pract-cl-guid-caring-v1.pdf)
- Your local social services can provide information about services available locally
- Check with your doctor for other local resources

PERSONAL ALARMS

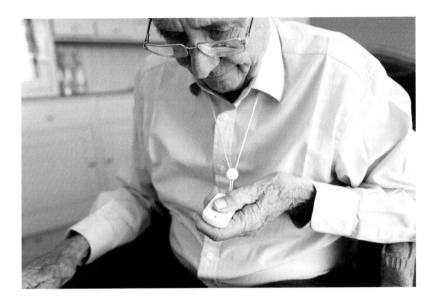

A personal alarm helps you to get help quickly in an emergency. It is worn on your hand or around your neck. When you press the button, you will be connected to someone for help.

You can find out more and buy a personal alarm through Age UK (https://www.ageuk.org.uk/products/ mobility-and-independence-at-home/ personal-alarms/).

OCCUPATIONAL THERAPY

Occupational therapists can help you improve your ability to do your everyday tasks if you are having any difficulty.

- They help you practise tasks in manageable stages.

- They can teach you different ways to complete the tasks.

- They will recommend changes to make the task easier.

- They can provide tools to make the task easier.

Your doctor, nurse or social care professionals can refer you to an occupational therapist.

EXAMPLES OF HELP THAT OCCUPATIONAL THERAPISTS CAN PROVIDE

- Help with tasks like preparing food, doing laundry or self-care

- Adapting your environment, for example by providing ramps for wheelchair access, a stairlift, rails for your bathroom or bedroom, toilet seats or shower seats

- Walking Aids

PHYSIOTHERAPY

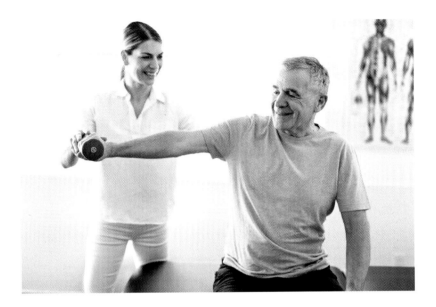

Physiotherapists will help you recover your movement and function if you have been injured or have come out of hospital after illness or surgery. They will help to prevent long-term disability.

HOUSING AND FINANCE

Where you live becomes increasingly important as you grow older, especially if you have long-term medical conditions. You need suitable accommodation that supports your physical and mental health needs.

- It enables you to stay safe, e.g. from falls or extreme weather.

- If you have limited mobility, everything needs to be accessible.

- Staying safe in a community helps prevent loneliness and social isolation.

Financial issues can affect your physical and mental health. In order to plan properly for your future, it may be helpful to get help from a financial adviser or your local Citizens Advice (https://www.citizensadvice.org.uk/).

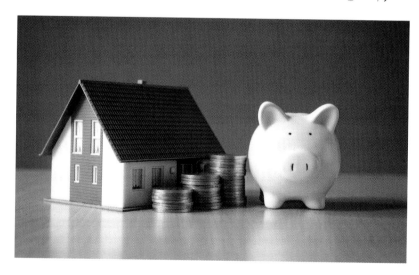

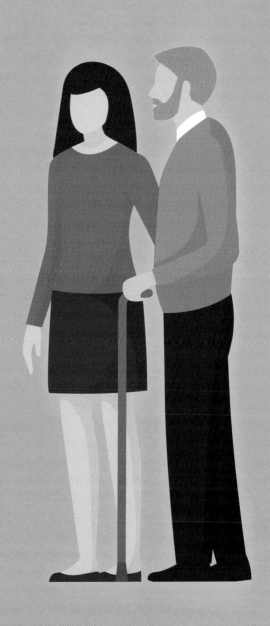

MENTAL CAPACITY ACT

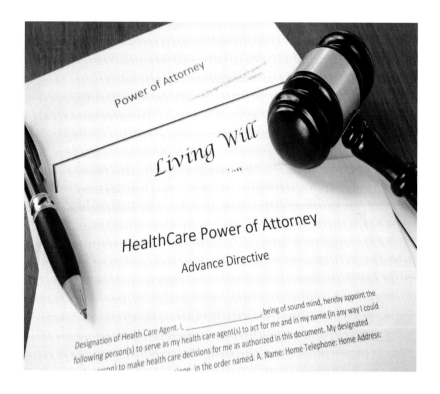

The Mental Capacity Act was introduced to protect people who lack capacity and enable good decisions to be made about their care or treatment.

WHAT MIGHT CAUSE ME TO LOSE CAPACITY?

Lack of capacity means when you are unable to make decisions for yourself. Lack of capacity is defined for a particular decision. Sometimes you can have the capacity to make certain decisions but not others.

This may develop slowly, with a progressive illness, such as dementia, or may happen suddenly with a medical emergency, such as a stroke. Examples of when you may lose capacity include:

- dementia

- brain injury

- stroke

- severe acute illness (physical/mental)

- severe learning disability.

THE FIVE PRINCIPLES OF THE MENTAL CAPACITY ACT

Health professionals assess your capacity on the following principles.

1. Assume that a person has the capacity to make a decision themselves unless it is proved otherwise.

2. Wherever possible, help people to make their own decisions.

3. Do not treat a person as lacking the capacity to make a decision just because they make an unwise decision

4. If you make a decision for someone who doesn't have the capacity, it must be in their best interests

5. Treatment and care provided to someone who lacks capacity should be the least restrictive of their basic rights and freedom.

HOW IS MENTAL CAPACITY ASSESSED FOR A SPECIFIC DECISION?

Mental capacity is assessed by asking questions to decide whether a person is able to make decisions for themselves. This is a sensitive issue and for big decisions, such as moving into care, it may need to be assessed on several occasions, perhaps at different times of the day or in different settings.

It is important that the person being assessed does not feel under pressure. If the time or place does not feel appropriate, it may be better to delay the decision until the person is better able to cope.

All the relevant information for the decision and any alternatives that are available should be provided, using simple language, and non-verbal communication if appropriate. It is usually helpful to have a trusted family member, carer or advocate to help frame the questions in an appropriate way.

The questions will focus on the ability to:

1. understand the information for a specific decision
2. retain the information
3. weigh up the information
4. express back the decision.

EXAMPLE

Mr Jones is an 82-year-old gentleman with dementia. He will need to be referred to have a camera test to check why he has developed anaemia.

He will need mental capacity assessment in this situation for this specific decision.

He will need to be told about the procedure in simple terms – what is involved in the procedure, the pros and cons if it is not done, and about possible complications.

Once this information is given, he has to understand the information and make a decision. He will need to be able to say why he has made a particular decision.

If he has any difficulty in understanding, making or expressing his decision, he will be said to lack capacity for this specific decision.

BEST INTEREST MEETING

If someone has been assessed as lacking capacity, best interest meeting can be arranged to help make a decision about that person's care or treatment. This usually involves a social worker and/or relevant clinicians, as well as any family member, carer or advocate who is involved.

The person is encouraged to attend if they are able, and it is thought to be appropriate. They will be asked if they have any objection to the attendance of anyone else who is there.

The patient's wishes, beliefs and feelings are considered in the discussion. Alternatives are considered, and a decision is made in the best interest of the patient. Any decision involves finding the least restrictive option that minimises interference with the patient's basic rights and freedom.

DEPRIVATION OF LIBERTY SAFEGUARDS (DOLS)

Deprivation of Liberty Safeguards is part of the Mental Capacity Act. They are safeguards put in place to make sure that people in hospital or residential care who have been assessed as lacking capacity are looked after in a way that does not cause harm.

Where a restriction is placed on a person who lacks capacity, it may be considered as deprivation of liberty and can be unlawful.

WHAT HAPPENS TO PROTECT THE INDIVIDUAL?

1. The patient lacks capacity and needs restriction.

2. The provider of care (hospital or care home) has to apply to the local authority to arrange for an assessment.

3. Assessment is done to check whether the deprivation is in the best interest of the individual:

YES:	NO:
legal authorization is given and a DOLS statement provided	the care and treatment package must be changed.

INDEPENDENT MENTAL CAPACITY ADVOCATE

When you lack the capacity to make decisions or you don't have any family or friends to make decisions for you regarding your care and well-being, you will have a choice to have an independent advocate (a person who can speak on your behalf) to help make the right choices for you. This will not cost you anything.

You can contact your doctor, social worker or local authority to get more information about locally available advocates.

USEFUL RESOURCES

- SeAp Advocacy – What is independent mental capacity advocacy? (https://www.seap.org.uk/services/independent-mental-capacity-advocacy/what-is-independent-mental-capacity-advocacy.html)

- POhWER – Independent mental health advocacy (https://www.pohwer.net/independent-mental-health-advocacy-imha)

- VoiceAbility – independent mental capacity advocacy (https://www.voiceability.org/about-advocacy/independent-mental-capacity-advocacy)

PLANNING AHEAD IN CASE YOU LOSE CAPACITY TO MAKE DECISIONS

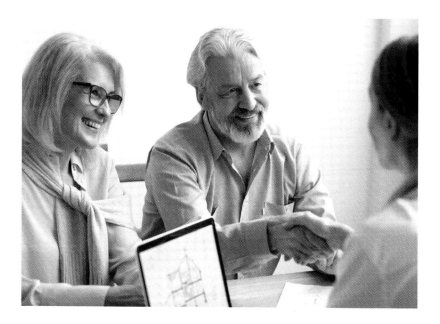

As you get older, it is a good idea to plan ahead and make your wishes known, in case you lose capacity to make decisions at a later stage. In addition to making a will for when you die, there are several ways you can help those who will care for you while you are still alive to understand what you would want if you were able to make your own decisions.

ADVANCE STATEMENTS

An advance statement is a statement you can write while you have mental capacity, about your wishes, beliefs, preferences and values regarding your future care if you no longer have mental capacity.

It is not legally binding but would be used when making best interest decisions.

Examples of what might be included are information about:

- your preferred place of care – home, hospital, nursing home or hospice
- your religious or spiritual beliefs
- your preferences for daily activities and self-care.

You can let your family, carers and/or clinicians know about it. You can ask your doctor to keep a copy on your medical notes.

You don't have to sign the statement, but it adds value if you do.

LIVING WILL (ALSO KNOWN AS ADVANCE DECISION, OR ADVANCE DECISION TO REFUSE TREATMENT)

A living will is a legally binding document that records your decision to refuse a specific treatment for a time in the future when you may lack the capacity to consent to or refuse that treatment.

It has the same effect as a decision made by a person with capacity, and health-care professionals must follow the decision.

It must state clearly that the decision applies even if your life is at risk and it must be in writing, signed and witnessed.

You can inform family members, carers or clinicians about your decision and ask to have a copy placed in your medical record.

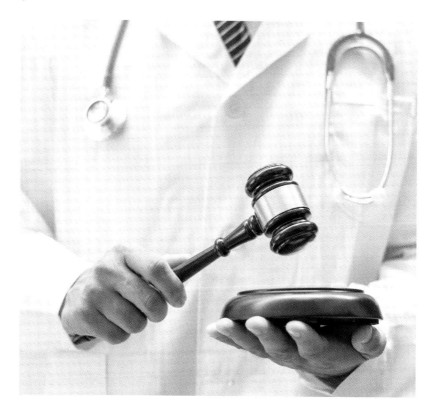

LASTING POWER OF ATTORNEY

Lasting Power of Attorney (previously known as Enduring Power of Attorney) is a legal document that enables you to give permission to another person (your attorney) to make decisions about your care and welfare.

It gives you control over what happens to you if you have an accident or illness that impairs your capacity to make decisions.

WHO CAN THAT PERSON BE?

You can appoint anyone that you trust as your attorney, or several people, and you can give them the power to act individually, or require that all attorneys have to agree with any decision. Most people appoint a trusted family member or members.

There are two types of Lasting Power of Attorney:

- Health and welfare – e.g. for decisions relating to self-care, medical care, moving to a care home and life-sustaining treatment

- Property and financial affairs – e.g. for managing your bank account, paying bills, collecting pension and benefits and selling your house.

MORE INFORMATION

Further information, forms and advice are available from The Office of the Public Guardian (0300 456 0300; https://www.gov.uk/government/organisations/office-of-the-public-guardian).

DO NOT ATTEMPT CARDIOPULMONARY RESUSCITATION – DNA-CPR

A DNA-CPR statement records that you should not be resuscitated (cardiopulmonary resuscitation) if your heart stops beating.

WHAT HAPPENS DURING CARDIOPULMONARY RESUSCITATION (CPR)?

- Compressions on your chest

- Artificial breathing

- Medications to revive your heart beat

- An Electric shock on your chest

WHAT HAPPENS IF CPR IS SUCCESSFUL?

- Once your heartbeat is restored, you may need hospital admission for continued treatment; this may mean that you will need to be in the intensive care unit and need a ventilator.

- There may be brain damage as a result of your brain not getting enough oxygen when your heart stopped beating. You may not recover the same brain function as before CPR.

- Your chances of recovery depend on your underlying health condition(s).

WHEN IS CPR NOT ATTEMPTED?

CPR will not be attempted if you have a severe underlying illness where recovery will lead to a poor outcome, or where there is likely to be severe brain damage.

CAN I BE INVOLVED IN MAKING THE DECISION?

Yes, you can make an advance decision after taking into consideration all the information.

WHO DECIDES NOT TO ATTEMPT CPR?

Clinicians involved in your care will usually make the decision. They will discuss this with you if you have the capacity. If not, a best interest decision is made. Your family and carers can be involved in the discussions.

This document is shared among all the health professionals, such as your doctors, nurses, ambulance team, and the out-of-hours care/palliative care team.

RECOMMENDED SUMMARY PLAN FOR EMERGENCY CARE AND TREATMENT (RESPECT)

ReSPECT is a process designed to encourage an informed and open discussion between patients and health professionals, with the aim of ensuring that decisions that need to be taken in an emergency situation reflect a person's own preferences and wishes.

USEFUL RESOURCES

- Dying Matters (www.dyingmatters.org)
- Compassion in Dying – Making decisions and planning your care (https://compassionindying.org.uk/making-decisions-and-planning-your-care)

BASIC LIFE SUPPORT

If you find anyone collapsed, you can attempt basic life support.

You can get formal training. Find out more from local first aid groups.

Steps in basic life support include:

1. Check if the person is unresponsive and whether or not they are breathing.

2. If there are no signs of breathing, call for help.

3. Perform 30 chest compressions.

4. If you are comfortable doing so, you can give 2 rescue breaths before continuing with another 30 chest compressions; if not, continue chest compressions until help arrives.

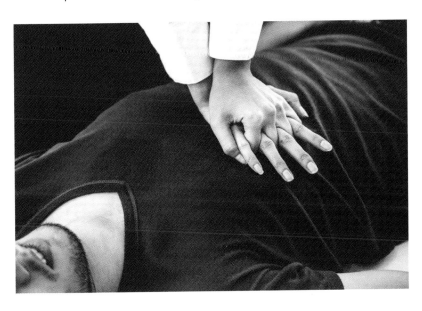

ORGAN DONATION

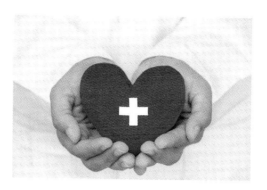

Organ donation involves donating your organs to some-one who needs a transplant, or for research purpose.

WHO CAN GIVE CONSENT?

There is no age limit on giving consent. A medical specialist will decide on the suitability of your organs at the time of your death. However, you cannot donate if you have Creutzfeldt Jakob disease (CJD), Ebola virus disease, active cancer, HIV or hepatitis C.

HOW DO I GIVE CONSENT?

You can register your consent by calling 0300 123 323, or online at www.organdonation.nhs.uk.

Note: The law is changing and, from Spring 2020, all adults in England will be considered to have given consent to be an organ donor when they die, unless they have recorded a decision not to donate or have one of the conditions listed above. You can find out more about opting out by calling 0300 303 2094, or on the NHS organ donation website given above.

END-OF-LIFE CARE

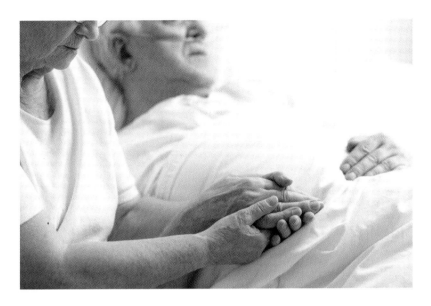

End-of-life care is support for people who are in the last days, weeks, months or years of their life.

WHEN IS END-OF-LIFE CARE REQUIRED?

End-of-life care may be used for the following:

- advanced incurable disease, like cancer, dementia, motor neurone disease

- multiple medical conditions and frailty, with a life expectancy of fewer than 12 months

- life-threatening acute illness with or without an underlying medical condition.

PLANNING END-OF-LIFE CARE

It is important for you and your family to plan your end-of-life-care:

- so that you can end your life according to your wishes, beliefs and preferences
- so that you can die with dignity
- to support your family, carers and others who are important to you.

Planning can take place wherever you are – in your home or care home, in a hospital or in a hospice.

Some or all of the following are likely to be involved in planning your care:

- doctors/nurses
- social care workers
- palliative care team
- occupational therapist
- physiotherapist
- religious adviser
- your family.

WHAT IS PALLIATIVE CARE?

If you have an incurable condition, you will receive palliative care to help cope with your symptoms. This is provided by a group of your doctors, specialist doctors, nurses and Macmillan team.

END-OF-LIFE CARE & LEGAL ASPECTS

The symptoms could be pain, nausea, vomiting, breathing difficulty and psychological symptoms.

EUTHANASIA

Euthanasia is a process of deliberating ending a person's life to relieve suffering. It is sometimes called mercy killing.

Assisted suicide is when a person deliberately assists or encourages another person to kill themselves.

Both are illegal in the UK and punishable by law.

The palliative care team will support you to relieve suffering during the end of your life or the life of someone you love.

USEFUL RESOURCES

- Dying Matters (http://help.dyingmatters.org/)
- You can also get more information from your doctor, nurse or palliative care team.

COPING WITH DEATH AND BEREAVEMENT

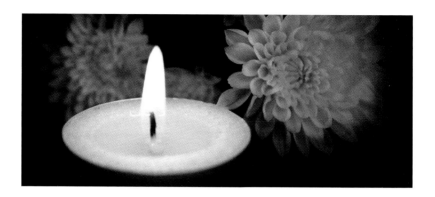

Bereavement is a feeling of grief after the death of some-one close to you. The natural period of grief is variable but is likely to be at least 1–2 years.

You may feel some or all of the following:

- sadness

- crying

- anger

- extreme tiredness

- guilt

- shock

- loneliness and feelings of social isolation.

HOW CAN I COPE WITH GRIEF?

Positive coping mechanisms

- Accepting that your feelings are normal

- Talking to family and friends whom you trust
- Talking to a bereavement counsellor or religious advisor
- Giving yourself time and engaging in other activities to keep you distracted

Negative coping mechanisms

- Alcohol
- Smoking
- Drugs

These have long-term side-effects and are likely to worsen the bereavement process.

HOW DO I KNOW IF I NEED HELP AND WHERE CAN I FIND IT?

If your emotions are affecting your daily activities, such as self-care and you are not eating, have a very low mood or thoughts of self-harm, you need to seek professional help from your doctor, who may refer you for counselling.

You could also seek help from:

- Cruse Bereavement Care (https://www.cruse.org.uk/; free helpline 0800808 1677)
- nidirect government services, which has useful information about what to do after a person dies, such as registering the death, dealing with finances, arranging a funeral, etc (www.nidirect.gov.uk/articles/what-do-when-someone-dies-checklist).

SOCIAL ISOLATION AND LONELINESS

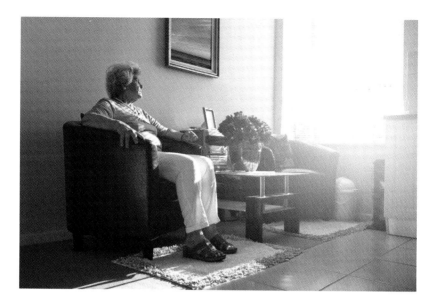

Lack of quality relationships with people around you can lead to negative emotions or sadness, owing to being lonely.

CAUSES OF LONELINESS

- Bereavement
- Lack of friends
- Poor physical health
- Living in a care home – far from family
- Financial difficulties

HEALTH EFFECTS OF LONELINESS

- Low mood

- Depression

- Anxiety

- Poor physical health

- Deterioration of chronic health conditions

HOW CAN I COMBAT LONELINESS?

- Group classes/activities

- Charity work

- Volunteering

- Looking after pets

- Using computers/phones to communicate with family and friends

- Exploring new hobbies

- Creating local hubs to transfer your skills to the younger generation

- Downsizing your house, so you live close to other older people – sheltered accommodation, retirement village, apartments

- The Silver Line helpline for older people (0800 470 8090; https://www.thesilverline.org.uk/)

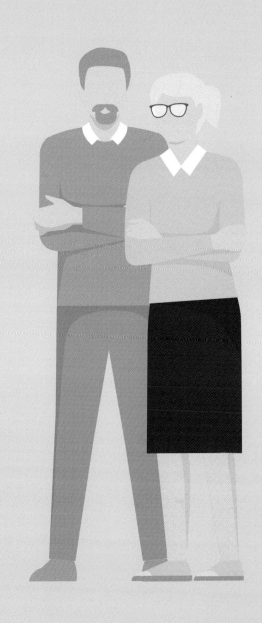

GOING TO SEE YOUR DOCTOR OR SPECIALIST

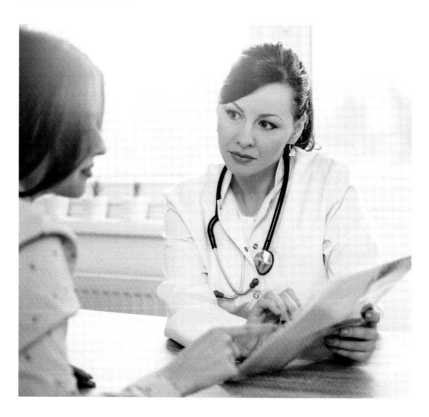

When you have an appointment with your doctor or hospital specialist, it is important that you are able to say all that you want to and get the information you need.

You may be anxious or upset about something and these emotions may make it difficult to remember to ask or discuss everything you wanted to.

In such situations, it would be helpful to write down beforehand the questions/topics you would like to discuss and take a notebook with you so you can write down anything important that the doctor tells you. It might also be helpful to take a trusted family member or friend with you, who can also listen to what is being said and remind you of anything you forgot.

Know beforehand how much time you have to spend with your doctor. Mention it to the receptionist if you think you will need to spend a bit longer to discuss your issues so that you don't feel rushed.

Ask the doctor or nurse for any leaflets or further information you can read.

Find out whether they can get more information from other specialists or whether you could come back to see the doctor or nurse for clarifications of any doubts.

HOSPITAL ADMISSION

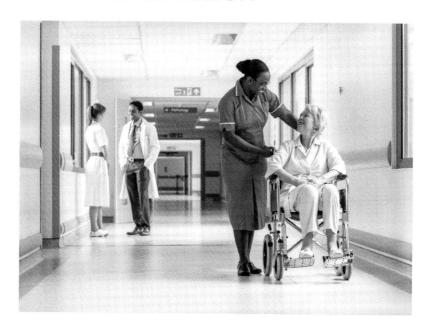

Being admitted to hospital can be a difficult experience, especially if it is for an emergency.

NON-EMERGENCY ADMISSION

If you know in advance that you're a going to be admitted to hospital, you have some time to plan and ask questions beforehand. Try to do the following:

- Make sure you know and understand why you are being admitted to hospital and what treatment and care you will have while you are there.

- Try to find out how long you are likely to be in the hospital for and what care you will need after you go home

- Ask questions about any complications or side-effects of your treatment

- Make sure your family and friends know you will be in the hospital, know when they can visit and can do anything you need at home.

EMERGENCY ADMISSION

- Being admitted to the hospital in an emergency can be quite a shock. It is important to trust that you will be well looked after and the health professionals in the hospital will give you the best care possible.

- It is helpful if you always know the contact details of one or two people you know to contact in an emergency. You can ask the hospital to contact them if you are not able to.

- You should always follow the instructions of the professionals who are looking after you and cooperate as best you can, to give them any information they need.

- You can discuss your concerns with the nurses or doctors who see you and express your wishes about how you want to be treated.

MEDICAL ERRORS OR NEGLIGENCE: HOW TO MAKE A COMPLAINT

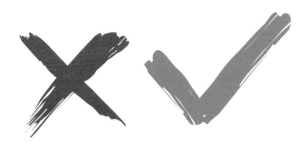

The way care is provided can be very complex, especially if you have several conditions, and it is not uncommon to come across medical errors. Many important lessons have been learnt from mistakes and the care provided for subsequent patients has improved, so it is important that you tell someone if your care was not good enough or mistakes were made.

There are many reasons why medical errors happen – e.g. tiredness, staff and system issues, incompetence, miscommunication, delay in treatment, poor policies, to name a few.

If a medical error occurs, it can be disabling and frustrating for both yourself and the health professionals involved. It can be a long process and can affect your general health.

An honest discussion with the relevant professionals and authorities about what happened can give you peace of mind as to why it happened.

You may need extra support from family/friends or counsellors during this period, to cope with the incident.

Your local doctors and hospitals will have a complaints policy, which you can access, and your local Patient Advice and Liaison Service (PALS) can help with lodging and investigating your complaint (https://www.nhs.uk/common-health-questions/nhs-services-and-treatments/what-is-pals-patient-advice-and-liaison-service/). Your doctor or hospital can give you the contact details of your nearest PALS office.

ALTERNATIVE AND COMPLEMENTARY THERAPIES

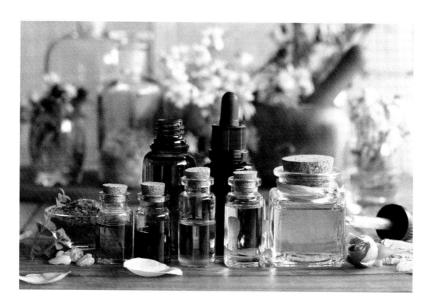

Alternative therapy is used instead of mainstream treatment and complementary therapy is used along with it.

Examples are:

- homoeopathy
- acupuncture
- osteopathy
- chiropractic
- herbal medicines.

It is up to you to find a reliable complementary and alternative medicine (CAM) practitioner and you will have to pay for their services. Osteopaths and chiropractors are regulated in the UK but not CAM practitioners.

Owing to the limited evidence available for these therapies, you need to find out about the treatment before starting, any side-effects, interactions with current medications, the duration of treatment, and proof of the practitioner's qualifications and references.

You need to be aware of some of the risks of these therapies:

- risks associated with buying medications online or by mail order

- fake medication

- substandard or contaminated medication

- unlicensed products that may contain banned or harmful substances.

The Medicines and Healthcare Regulatory Agency of the UK have published a list of banned and restricted herbal ingredients. You can find it at (https://www.gov.uk/government/publications/list-of-banned-or-restricted-herbal-ingredients-for-medicinal-use/banned-and-restricted-herbal-ingredients).

TRAVELLING WITH LONG-TERM MEDICAL CONDITIONS

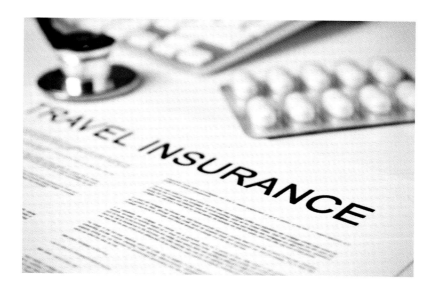

Travelling with a long-term medical condition can present some challenges, but if you plan ahead, they can usually be overcome.

- Make sure you have travel insurance.

- Discuss with your doctor or pharmacist regarding your medications to take and ensuring you have enough to last you while you are away.

- Speak to your doctor regarding your risk of DVT (clot in the legs) and any special measures like flight socks, medications to take and exercises to do.

- Make sure you have enough sun protection, depending on your skin type.

- Check regarding travel vaccinations and any outbreaks of diseases in the country you are travelling to.

USEFUL RESOURCES

- TravelHealthPro (www.travelhealthpro.org.uk)
- fitfortravel (www.fitfortravel.nhs.uk)
- NHS website – search for 'Travel' (www.nhs.uk)
- Patient – Health advice for travel abroad (https://patient.info/travel-and-vaccinations/health-advice-for-travel-abroad)

TECHNOLOGY

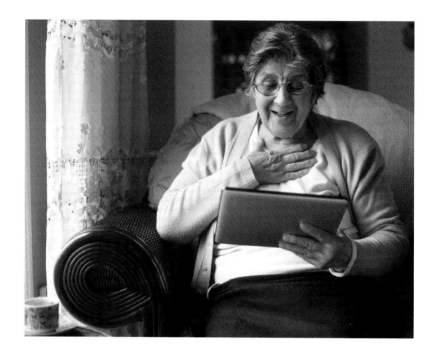

Learning to use the latest technology can be a daunting and long process but there are many benefits to it. Local libraries or charities can help you with the learning process. Learning from family members or friends can be another option.

Different technologies that can be used to help with your general health, in all sorts of ways, are:

- smartphone
- tablet

- computer – browsing the internet, email (for keeping in touch with family and friends), and online communities.

- video call to keep in touch with family and friends

- using various apps for hobbies and to plan and navigate car journeys

- using online pharmacy and doctors' services

- personal alarms.

PERSONAL MEDICAL LOG BOOK

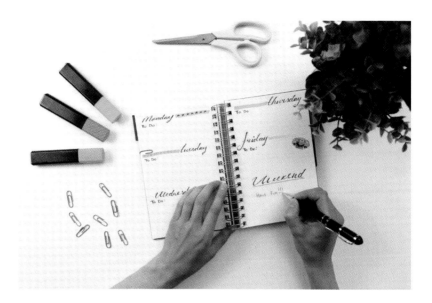

If you have one or more long-term medical conditions, it is a good idea to keep a personal medical log book so that all your health information is in one place.

Suggestions for items to include are:

- health conditions – medical, any surgeries/hospital admissions

- symptoms tracker

- family history

- physical health – pulse, blood pressure, height, weight, BMI

- food diary

- exercise diary

- mood chart
- pain diary
- smoking
- alcohol intake
- medications you are taking – special instructions for taking the medication and review follow-up date(s)
- allergies and medical alerts
- immunisations
- doctors, pharmacist, specialists and hospital contact numbers
- emergency numbers
- details of next of kin/family/friend(s)
- summary of any advance statement or advance decision document(s).